Keto Diet Cookbook

Over 50 Nutritional And Healthy Recipes For Beginners

Lucy Miles

TABLE OF CONTENTS

INTRODUCTION

Thank you for buying this cookbook! Now you will no longer have problems of imagination in the kitchen. Thanks to our recipes you can surprise your friends with always new and tasty dishes. With the nutritional information contained in each recipe, you can follow a balanced diet according to your needs. Have you ever gone to a restaurant to eat a specific dish? This cookbook will allow you to make some of your favorites at home. Cooking is an art that allows you to involve the whole family, so as well as satisfying the palate you have a good excuse to spend more time with the people you care about most. Choose your dish and have fun.

BREAKFAST RECIPES

01. Cheesy Ham Souffle

Serves: 4

Prep Time: 30 mins

Ingredients

- 1 cup cheddar cheese, shredded
- ½ cup heavy cream
- 6 large eggs
- 6 ounces ham, diced
- Salt and black pepper, to taste

Directions

1. Preheat the oven to 3500F and grease 4 ramekins gently.
2. Whisk together eggs in a medium bowl and add all other ingredients.
3. Mix well and pour the mixture into the ramekins.
4. Transfer into the ramekins and bake for about 18 minutes.
5. Remove from the oven and allow to slightly cool and serve.

Nutrition Amount per serving

Calories 342

Total Fat 26g 33%

Saturated Fat 13g 65%

Cholesterol 353mg 118%

Sodium 841mg 37%

Total Carbohydrate 3g 1%

Dietary Fiber 0.6g 2%

Total Sugars 0.8g

Protein 23.8g

02. Browned Butter Pumpkin Latte

Serves: 2

Prep Time: 10 mins

Ingredients

- 2 shots espresso
- 2 tablespoons butter
- 2 scoops Stevia
- 2 cups hot almond milk
- 4 tablespoons pumpkin puree

Directions

1. Heat butter on low heat in a small pan and allow to lightly brown.
2. Brew two shots of espresso and stir in the Stevia.
3. Add browned butter along with pumpkin puree and hot almond milk.
4. Blend for about 10 seconds on high and pour into 2 cups to serve.

Nutrition Amount per serving

Calories 227

Total Fat 22.6g 29%

Saturated Fat 18.3g 92%

Cholesterol 31mg 10%

Sodium 93mg 4%

Total Carbohydrate 4.5g 2%

Dietary Fiber 0.9g 3%

Total Sugars 1g, Protein 1.5g

03. Cauliflower Toast with Avocado

Serves: 2

Prep Time: 20 mins

Ingredients

- 1 large egg
- 1 small head cauliflower, grated
- 1 medium avocado, pitted and chopped
- ¾ cup mozzarella cheese, shredded
- Salt and black pepper, to taste

Directions

1. Preheat the oven to 420°F and line a baking sheet with parchment.
2. Place the cauliflower in a microwave safe bowl and microwave for about 7 minutes on high.
3. Spread on paper towels to drain after the cauliflower has completely cooled and press with a clean towel to remove excess moisture.
4. Put the cauliflower back in the bowl and stir in the mozzarella cheese and egg.
5. Season with salt and black pepper and stir until well combined.
6. Spoon the mixture onto the baking sheet in two rounded squares, as evenly as possible.
7. Bake for about 20 minutes until golden brown on the edges.

8. Mash the avocado with a pinch of salt and black pepper.
9. Spread the avocado onto the cauliflower toast and serve.

Nutrition Amount per serving

Calories 127

Total Fat 7g 9%

Saturated Fat 2.4g 12%

Cholesterol 99mg 33%

Sodium 139mg 6%

Total Carbohydrate 9.1g 3%

Dietary Fiber 4.8g 17%

Total Sugars 3.4g

Protein 9.3g

04. Breakfast Cheesy Sausage

Serves: 1

Prep Time: 20 mins

Ingredients

- 1 pork sausage link, cut open and casing discarded
- Sea salt and black pepper, to taste
- ¼ teaspoon thyme
- ¼ teaspoon sage
- ½ cup mozzarella cheese, shredded

Directions

1. Mix sausage meat with thyme, sage, mozzarella cheese, sea salt and black pepper.
2. Shape the mixture into a patty and transfer to a hot pan.
3. Cook for about 5 minutes per side and dish out to serve.

Nutrition Amount per serving

Calories 91

Total Fat 7.1g 9%

Saturated Fat 3g 15%

Cholesterol 17mg 6%

Sodium 218mg 9%

Total Carbohydrate 1.1g

Dietary Fiber 0.2g 1%

Total Sugars 0.2g

05. Keto Avocado Toast

Serves: 2

Prep Time: 20 mins

Ingredients

- 2 tablespoons sunflower oil
- ½ cup parmesan cheese, shredded
- 1 medium avocado, sliced
- Sea salt, to taste
- 4 slices cauliflower bread

Directions

1. Heat oil in a pan and cook cauliflower bread slices for about 2 minutes per side.
2. Season avocado with sea salt and place on the cauliflower bread.
3. Top with parmesan cheese and microwave for about 2 minutes.

Nutrition Amount per serving

Calories 141

Total Fat 10g 13%

Saturated Fat 4.6g 23%

Cholesterol 20mg 7%

Sodium 385mg 17%

Total Carbohydrate 4.5g 2%

Dietary Fiber 2.4g 9%

Total Sugars 0.7g

Protein 10.6g

06. Cream Cheese and Chive Fold-Overs

Serves: 2

Prep Time: 15 mins

Ingredients

- 6 tablespoons cream cheese
- 1 teaspoon lemon juice
- 4 coconut flour tortillas
- 3 tablespoons fresh chives, chopped
- 4 teaspoons olive oil

Directions

1. Whisk cream cheese thoroughly in a bowl and stir in chives and lemon juice.
2. Spread the cream cheese mixture evenly over the tortillas and fold into half-moon shapes.
3. Heat quarter of oil over medium high heat in a skillet and add a tortilla.
4. Cook until browned on both sides and repeat with the remaining tortillas.
5. Serve warm.

Nutrition Amount per serving

Calories 158

Total Fat 11.5g 15%

Saturated Fat 5g 25%

Cholesterol 17mg 6%

Sodium 45mg 2%

Total Carbohydrate 11.2g 4%

Dietary Fiber 6.5g 23%

Total Sugars 0.1g

Protein 3.4g

07. Chocolate Chip Waffles

Serves: 2

Prep Time: 30 mins

Ingredients

- 2 scoops vanilla protein powder
- 1 pinch pink Himalayan sea salt
- 50 grams sugar free chocolate chips
- 2 large eggs, separated
- 2 tablespoons butter, melted

Directions

1. Mix together egg yolks, vanilla protein powder and butter in a bowl.
2. Whisk together egg whites thoroughly in another bowl and transfer to the egg yolks mixture.
3. Add the sugar free chocolate chips and a pinch of pink salt.
4. Transfer this mixture in the waffle maker and cook according to manufacturer's instructions.

Nutrition Amount per serving

Calories 301

Total Fat 18.8g 24%

Saturated Fat 9.7g 49%

Cholesterol 229mg 76%

Sodium 242mg 11%

Total Carbohydrate 6.9g 3%

Dietary Fiber 1.3g 4%

Total Sugars 1.4g

08. Low Carb Cereal

Serves: 2

Prep Time: 25 mins

Ingredients

- 2 tablespoons flaxseeds
- ¼ cup almonds, slivered
- 1 tablespoon chia seeds
- 1½ cups almond milk, unsweetened
- 10 grams cocoa nibs

Directions

1. Mix together flaxseeds, almonds, chia seeds and cocoa nibs in a bowl.
2. Top with the almond milk and serve.

Nutrition Amount per serving

Calories 244

Total Fat 20.6g 26%

Saturated Fat 10.4g 52%

Cholesterol 0mg 0%

Sodium 11mg 0%

Total Carbohydrate 9.8g 4%

Dietary Fiber 6.5g 23%

Total Sugars 1.9g

09. Low Carb Detox Tea

Serves: 1

Prep Time: 10 mins

Ingredients

- 2 tablespoons apple cider vinegar
- 1 scoop Stevia
- 1 cup water
- 2 tablespoons lemon juice
- 1 teaspoon cinnamon

Directions

1. Boil water and add remaining ingredients.
2. Pour into a cup and serve hot.

Nutrition Amount per serving

Calories 19

Total Fat 0.3g 0%

Saturated Fat 0.3g 1%

Cholesterol 0mg 0%

Sodium 15mg 1%

Total Carbohydrate 2.8g 1%

Dietary Fiber 1.3g 5%

Total Sugars 0.8g

Protein 0.3g

10. Iced Matcha Latte

Serves: 1

Prep Time: 10 mins

Ingredients

- 1 tablespoon coconut oil
- 1 cup unsweetened cashew milk
- 1 teaspoon matcha powder
- 2 ice cubes
- 1/8 teaspoon vanilla bean

Directions

1. Mix together all the ingredients in a blender and blend until smooth.
2. Pour into a glass to serve.

Nutrition Amount per serving

Calories 161

Total Fat 16g 21%

Saturated Fat 12g 60%

Cholesterol 3mg 1%

Sodium 166mg 7%

Total Carbohydrate 2.9g 1%

Dietary Fiber 2g 7%

Total Sugars 1.4g

Protein 2.4

CHAFFLE RECIPES

01. Scrambled Egg Stuffed Chaffles

Preparation Time: 15 minutes Cooking Time: 28 minutes Servings: 4

Ingredients:

For the chaffles:

- 1 cup finely grated cheddar cheese
- 2 eggs, beaten

For the egg stuffing:

- 1 tbsp olive oil
- 4 large eggs
- 1 small green bell pepper, deseeded and chopped

- 1 small red bell pepper, deseeded and chopped
- Salt and freshly ground black pepper to taste
- 2 tbsp grated Parmesan cheese

Directions:

For the chaffles:

1. Preheat the waffle iron.
2. In a medium bowl, mix the cheddar cheese

and egg.

3. Open the iron, pour in a quarter of the mixture, close, and cook until crispy, 6 to 7 minutes.

4. Plate and make three more chaffles using the remaining mixture.

For the egg stuffing:

1. Meanwhile, heat the olive oil in a medium skillet over medium heat on a stovetop.

2. In a medium bowl, beat the eggs with the bell peppers, salt, black pepper, and Parmesan cheese.

3. Pour the mixture into the skillet and scramble until set to your likeness, 2 minutes.

4. Between two chaffles, spoon half of the scrambled eggs and repeat with the second set of chaffles.

5. Serve afterward.

Nutrition: Calories 387 Fats 22.52g Carbs 18.12g Net Carbs 17.52g Protein 27.76g

02. Mixed Berry- Vanilla Chaffles

Preparation Time: 10 minutes Cooking Time: 28 minutes Servings: 4

Ingredients:

- 1 egg, beaten
- ½ cup finely grated mozzarella cheese
- 1 tbsp cream cheese, softened
- 1 tbsp sugar-free maple syrup
- 2 strawberries, sliced
- 2 raspberries, slices
- ¼ tsp blackberry extract
- ¼ tsp vanilla extract
- ½ cup plain yogurt for serving

Directions:

1. Preheat the waffle iron.
2. In a medium bowl, mix all the ingredients except the yogurt.
3. Open the iron, lightly grease with cooking spray

and pour in a quarter of the mixture.

4. Close the iron and cook until golden brown and crispy, 7 minutes.
5. Remove the chaffle onto a plate and set aside.
6. Make three more chaffles with the remaining mixture.
7. To Servings: top with the yogurt and enjoy.

Nutrition: Calories 78 Fats 5.29g Carbs 3.02g Net Carbs 2.72g Protein 4.32g

03. Chaffles with Vanilla Sauce

Serving: 6-8 chaffles (6-1/2 inches).

Preparation Time: 15 minutes Cooking Time: 30 minutes

Ingredients

- 1-2/3 cups all-purpose flour
- 4 teaspoons baking powder
- 1/2 teaspoon salt
- 2 eggs, separated
- 3-2/3 cups milk, divided
- 6 tablespoons canola oil
- 1/2 cup sugar
- 1 teaspoon vanilla extract
- 1/2 cup mozzarella cheese, shredded
- Fresh strawberries

Direction

1. In a bowl, combine flour, baking powder and salt. In another bowl, beat egg yolks lightly. Add 1-2/3 cups milk and oil; stir into dry

Ingredients just until moistened. Set aside 1/4 cup batter in a small bowl. Beat egg whites until stiff peaks form; fold into remaining batter. Add mozzarella cheese and stir well.

2. Bake in a preheated waffle iron according to manufacturer's directions until golden brown. In a saucepan, heat sugar and remaining milk until scalded. Stir a small amount into reserved batter; return all to pan. Bring to a boil; boil for 5- 7 minutes or until thickened. Remove from the heat; add vanilla and mix well (sauce will thicken upon standing). Serve over chaffles. Top with berries.

Nutrition: Calories: 429 calories Total Fat: 21g Cholesterol: 91mg Sodium: 558mg Total Carbohydrate: 50g Protein: 11g Fiber: 1g

04. Pecan Pumpkin Chaffle

Preparation Time: 15 minutes Servings: 2

Ingredients:

- 1 egg
- 2 tbsp pecans, toasted and chopped
- 2 tbsp almond flour
- 1 tsp erythritol
- 1/4 tsp pumpkin pie spice
- 1 tbsp pumpkin puree
- 1/2 cup mozzarella cheese, grated

Directions:

1. Preheat your waffle maker.
2. Beat egg in a small bowl.
3. Add remaining ingredients and mix well.
4. Spray waffle maker with cooking spray.
5. Pour half batter in the hot waffle maker and **cook**

for 5 minutes or until golden brown. Repeat with the remaining batter.

6. Serve and enjoy.

Nutrition: Calories 121 Fat 9.7 g Carbohydrates 5.7 g Sugar 3.3 g Protein 6.7 g Cholesterol 86 mg

05. Quick & Easy Blueberry Chaffle

Preparation Time: 15 minutes Servings: 2

Ingredients:

- 1 egg, lightly beaten
- 1/4 cup blueberries
- 1/2 tsp vanilla
- 1 oz cream cheese
- 1/4 tsp baking powder, gluten-free
- 4 tsp Swerve
- 1 tbsp coconut flour

Directions:

1. Preheat your waffle maker.
2. In a small bowl, mix coconut flour, baking powder, and Swerve until well combined.
3. Add vanilla, cream cheese, egg, and vanilla and whisk until combined.
4. Spray waffle maker with cooking spray.

5. Pour half batter in the hot waffle maker and top with 4-5 blueberries and cook for 4-5 minutes until golden brown. Repeat with the remaining batter.

6. Serve and enjoy.

Nutrition: Calories 135, Fat 8.2 g, Carbohydrates 11 g Sugar 2.6 g, Protein 5 g, Cholesterol 97 mg

06. Apple Cinnamon Chaffles

Preparation Time: 20 minutes Servings: 3

Ingredients:

- 3 eggs, lightly beaten
- 1 cup mozzarella cheese, shredded
- ¼ cup apple, chopped
- ½ tsp monk fruit sweetener
- 1 ½ tsp cinnamon
- ¼ tsp baking powder, gluten- free
- 2 tbsp coconut flour

Directions:

1. Preheat your waffle maker.
2. Add eggs in a mixing bowl and beat until frothy.
3. Add remaining ingredients and stir until well combined.
4. Spray waffle maker with cooking spray.
5. Pour 1/3 of batter in the hot waffle maker and

cook for 4 minutes or until golden brown. Repeat with the remaining batter.

6. Serve and enjoy.

Nutrition: Calories 142 Fat 7.4 g
Carbohydrates 9.7 g Sugar 3 g
Protein 9.6 g Cholesterol 169 mg

07. Mozzarella Peanut Butter Chaffle

Preparation Time: 15 minutes Servings: 2

Ingredients:

- 1 egg, lightly beaten
- 2 tbsp peanut butter
- 2 tbsp Swerve
- 1/2 cup mozzarella cheese, shredded

Directions:

1. Preheat your waffle maker.
2. In a bowl, mix egg, cheese, Swerve, and peanut butter until well combined.
3. Spray waffle maker with cooking spray.
4. Pour half batter in the hot waffle maker and cook for 4 minutes or until golden brown. Repeat with the remaining batter.
5. Serve and enjoy.

Nutrition: Calories 150 Fat 11.5 g
Carbohydrates 5.6 g Sugar 1.7 g
Protein 8.8 g Cholesterol 86 mg

08. Sweet Vanilla Chocolate Chaffle

Preparation Time: 10 minutes Servings: 1

Ingredients:

- 1 egg, lightly beaten
- 1/4 tsp cinnamon
- 1/2 tsp vanilla
- 1 tbsp Swerve
- 2 tsp unsweetened cocoa powder
- 1 tbsp coconut flour
- 2 oz cream cheese, softened

Directions:

1. Add all ingredients into the small bowl and mix until well combined.
2. Spray waffle maker with cooking spray.
3. Pour batter in the hot waffle maker and cook until golden brown.
4. Serve and enjoy.

Nutrition: Calories 312 Fat 25.4 g Carbohydrates 11.5 g Sugar 0.8 g Protein 11.6 g Cholesterol 226 mg

09. Peanut Butter Sandwich Chaffle

Preparation Time: 15 minutes Servings: 1

For chaffle:

- 1 egg, lightly beaten
- 1/2 cup mozzarella cheese, shredded
- 1/4 tsp espresso powder
- 1 tbsp unsweetened chocolate chips
- 1 tbsp Swerve
- 2 tbsp unsweetened cocoa powder
-

For filling:

- 1 tbsp butter, softened
- 2 tbsp Swerve
- 3 tbsp creamy peanut butter

Directions:

1. Preheat your waffle maker.

2. In a bowl, whisk together egg, espresso powder, chocolate chips, Swerve, and cocoa powder.

3. Add mozzarella cheese and stir well.
4. Spray waffle maker with cooking spray.

5. Pour 1/2 of the batter in the hot waffle maker and cook for 3-4 minutes or until golden brown. Repeat with the remaining batter.

***For filling*:**

1. In a small bowl, stir together butter, Swerve, and peanut butter until smooth.

2. Once chaffles is cool, then spread filling mixture between two chaffle and place in the fridge for 10 minutes.

3. Cut chaffle sandwich in half and serve.

Nutrition: Calories 190 Fat 16.1 g
Carbohydrates 9.6 g Sugar 1.1 g
Protein 8.2 g Cholesterol 101 mg

10. Cherry Chocolate Chaffle

Ingredients:

- 1 egg, lightly beaten
- 1 tbsp unsweetened chocolate chips
- 2 tbsp sugar-free cherry pie filling
- 2 tbsp heavy whipping cream
- 1/2 cup mozzarella cheese, shredded
- 1/2 tsp baking powder, gluten-free
- 1 tbsp Swerve
- 1 tbsp unsweetened cocoa powder
- 1 tbsp almond flour

Directions:

1. Preheat the waffle maker.
2. In a bowl, whisk together egg, cheese, baking powder, Swerve, cocoa powder, and almond flour.
3. Spray waffle maker with cooking spray.

4. Pour batter in the hot waffle maker and cook until golden brown.

5. Top with cherry pie filling, heavy whipping cream, and chocolate chips and serve.

Nutrition: Calories 264 Fat 22 g
Carbohydrates 8.5 g Sugar 0.5 g
Protein 12.7 g Cholesterol 212 mg

11. Pulled Pork Chaffle Sandwiches

Preparation Time: 20 minutes Cooking Time: 28 minutes Servings: 4

Ingredients:

- **2 eggs, beaten**
- **1 cup finely grated cheddar cheese**
-
- **¼ tsp baking powder**
- **2 cups cooked and shredded pork**
- **1 tbsp sugar-free BBQ sauce**
- **2 cups shredded coleslaw mix**
- **2 tbsp apple cider vinegar**
- **½ tsp salt**
- **¼ cup ranch dressing**

Directions:

1. Preheat the waffle iron.
2. In a medium bowl, mix the eggs, cheddar cheese, and baking powder.
3. Open the iron and add a quarter of the mixture. Close and cook until crispy, 7 minutes.
4. Transfer the chaffle to a plate and make 3 more chaffles in the same manner.
5. Meanwhile, in another medium bowl, mix the pulled pork with the BBQ sauce until well combined. Set aside.
6. Also, mix the coleslaw mix, apple cider vinegar, salt, and ranch dressing in another medium bowl.
7. When the chaffles are ready, on two pieces, divide the pork and then top with the ranch coleslaw. Cover with the remaining chaffles and insert mini skewers to secure the sandwiches.
8. Enjoy afterward.

Nutrition: Calories 374 Fats 23.61g Carbs 8.2g Net Carbs 8.2g Protein 28.05g

SOUP, STEWS, BROTHS & SAUCES

01. Creamy Garlic Chicken Soup

Servings: 4

Preparation time: 10 minutes

Cooking Time: 5-10 minutes

INGREDIENTS

- 2 tablespoons butter
- 4 ounces cream cheese, cubed
- 14.5-ounce chicken broth
- 2 cups chicken, shredded
- ¼ cup heavy cream
- 2 tablespoons Stacey Hawkins Garlic Gusto Seasoning
- Salt, to taste

DIRECTIONS

1. Take a saucepan and place it over medium heat.
2. Add butter into the saucepan and melt the butter.
3. Put shredded chicken to pan and coat with melted butter.
4. Add cream cheese and Stacey Hawkins garlic gusto seasoning when chicken is warm.
5. Mix to blend the Ingredients.
6. Add chicken broth, heavy cream and evenly distributed cream cheese.

7. Bring them to boil then reduce the heat to low.
8. Simmer for 3-4 minutes.
9. Add salt to taste and serve.
10. Enjoy!

NUTRITION: Calories:307;Total Fat:25g; Protein: 16g; Carbs: 2g

02. Leftover Turkey Stew

Servings: 12

Preparation time: 10 minutes
Cooking Time: 25 minutes

INGREDIENTS

- 15 ounces can vegetables, mixed
- 2 cups turkey, cooked and cubed
- 14 ounces can chicken broth
- 3 tablespoon butter

DIRECTIONS

1. Take a saucepan and put all the Ingredients into it.
2. Bring it to boil.
3. Reduce the heat to low.
4. Simmer for about 25 minutes.
5. Dish out and serve hot.
6. Enjoy!

NUTRITION:

Calories: 143;
Total Fat: 6.8g;
Protein: 16.2g;
Carbs: 3.4g

03. Cheesy Beef Sausage Soup

Servings: 16

Preparation time: 30 minutes

Cooking Time: 6 hours

INGREDIENTS

- 12 ounces beer
- 14 ounces of beef smoked sausage, chopped
- 1 cup heavy cream
- 8 ounces cream cheese
- 1 teaspoon of sea salt
- ½ teaspoon black pepper
- 1 teaspoon red pepper flakes
- 32 ounces beef stock
- 2 cups sharp cheddar cheese, shredded
- 1 onion, diced
- 4 garlic cloves, minced
- 1 cup celery, chopped
- 1 cup carrots, chopped

DIRECTIONS

1. Turn on your slow cooker and add all the Ingredients except cheese and cream into it.
2. Mix them well.
3. Cover the lid.

4. Cook for 4 hours on low.
5. Now whisk in the cheese and cream.
6. Cook covered for 2 hours more.
7. Serve and enjoy!

NUTRITION:
Calories:244;
Total Fat:17g;
Protein: 5g;
Carbs: 4g

04. Creamy Subtle Broccoli Soup

Servings: 3

Preparation time:

5 minutes

Cooking Time:

35 minutes

INGREDIENTS

- 3 cups broccoli florets, chopped
- 1 can full-fat coconut milk
- ½ teaspoon onion powder
- 3 cups celery, chopped
- 2 cups vegetable stock
- ½ teaspoon garlic powder
- Red pepper flakes as needed
- Salt and pepper, to taste

DIRECTIONS

1. Take a pot and place it over medium heat.
2. Add the Ingredients to the pot.
3. Cook for about 30 minutes until the broccoli and celery are soft.
4. Transfer the soup to a blender and process them until smooth.
5. Serve hot and enjoy!

NUTRITION: Calories:200;TotalFat:17g; Protein: 4g; Carbs: 5g

05. Melon Soup

Servings: 4

Preparation time: 6 minutes

INGREDIENTS

- 4 cups casaba melon, seeded and cubed
- 1 tablespoon fresh ginger, grated
- ¾ cup of coconut milk
- Juice of 2 lime
- Salt as needed

DIRECTIONS

1. Add the lime juice, coconut milk, casaba melon, ginger and salt into your blender.
2. Blend it for 1-2 minutes until you get a smooth mixture.
3. Serve and enjoy!

NUTRITION: Calories: 134; Total Fat: 9g; Protein: 2g; Carbs: 13g

VEGANS & VEGETARIANS

01. Sesame Shrimp Bites

Preparation Time: 15 minutes

Servings 6

NUTRITION: 107 Calories; 4.9g Fat; 1g Carbs; 15.3g Protein; 0.8g Fiber

INGREDIENTS

- 1 pound shrimp, deveined and shelled
- 2 tablespoons sesame seeds
- 1/4 cup fish stock
- 2 garlic cloves, pressed
- 2 tablespoons sesame oil
- 1/2 cup onions, chopped
- 1 teaspoon chili powder
- 2 tablespoons dry white wine
- Salt and ground black pepper, to taste

DIRECTIONS

1. Heat the oil in a saucepan over a moderately-high heat. Cook the shrimp, garlic and onions for about 3 minutes.
2. Add in the remaining Nutritional Info per Serving: and cook for 10 minutes more until cooked through.
3. Storing
4. Place the shrimp in airtight containers or Ziploc bags; keep in your refrigerator for up 3 to 4 days.
5. For freezing, arrange cooked shrimp in a single layer on a baking tray; place in your freezer for about 15 minutes, or until it begins to harden.
6. Transfer the frozen shrimp to heavy-duty freezer bags. Freeze up to 3 months. Defrost in your refrigerator. Enjoy!

02. Easy Turkey Bites with Spicy Sauce

Preparation Time: 30 minutes

Servings 8

NUTRITION: 153 Calories; 6.7g Fat; 4.6g Carbs; 21.8g Protein; 0.7g Fiber

INGREDIENTS

- 1/3 cup flax meal
- 3/4 cup almond flour
- 2 eggs, whisked
- 1 ¼ pounds turkey tenderloin, cut into 20 pieces
- Salt and black pepper, to season

For the Sauce:

- 1/2 tablespoon Sriracha sauce
- 1/2 teaspoon cayenne pepper
- 1 teaspoon deli mustard
- 1 teaspoon garlic powder
- 1/3 cup tomato paste
- 1/3 teaspoon cumin

DIRECTIONS

1. Start by preheating your oven to 365 degrees F. Brush the bottom of a baking pan with cooking spray.
2. Toss the turkey pieces with salt and pepper. Mix the flax meal with the almond meal.
3. Dip the turkey pieces in the whisked egg, then, coat them with the meal mixture. Bake for 25 to 28 minutes.
4. Whisk all the sauce Nutritional Info per Serving: and reserve.
5. Storing
6. Wrap the turkey pieces in foil before packing them into an airtight container; keep in your refrigerator for up to 3 to 4 days.
7. For freezing, place them in airtight containers or heavy-duty freezer bags.

   Freeze up to 2 to 3 months. Defrost in the refrigerator.
8. Place the sauce in airtight containers or Ziploc bags; keep in your refrigerator for up 3 to 4 days.
9. To freeze, place the sauce in separate Ziploc

bags and freeze up to 3 months. To defrost, place in your microwave for a few minutes. Bon appétit!

03. Spicy Parm Meatballs

Preparation Time: 15 minutes

Servings 10

NUTRITION: 158 Calories; 7.9g Fat; 0.4g Carbs; 20.4g Protein; 0.1g Fiber

INGREDIENTS

- 1 egg, beaten
- 1⁄3 cup double cream
- 3/4 pound ground turkey
- 1/2 pound ground pork
- 2 garlic cloves, finely minced
- 1 teaspoon shallot powder
- 1/2 teaspoon mustard seeds
- 1 teaspoon hot sauce
- 1/4 cup pork rinds, crushed
- 1/3 cup Parmesan cheese, grated
- Sea salt and black pepper, to taste
- 1 teaspoon fresh basil, minced

DIRECTIONS

1 In a mixing bowl, combine all Nutritional Info per Serving: until everything is well incorporated. Roll the mixture into small balls and arrange them on a parchment- lined baking sheet.
2 Bake in the preheated oven at 390 degrees F for 8 to 10 minutes. Then, flip them over and cook another 8 minutes until they are browned and slightly crisp on top.
3 Storing
4 Place the meatballs in airtight containers or Ziploc bags; keep in your refrigerator for up to 3 to 4 days.
    1. Freeze the meatballs in airtight containers or heavy-duty freezer bags. Freeze up to 3 to 4 months. To defrost, slowly reheat in a saucepan. Bon appétit!

04. Classic Cheese and Artichoke Dip

Preparation Time: 5 minutes

Servings 8

NUTRITION: 157 Calories; 11g Fat; 5.9g Carbs; 6.5g Protein; 2.7g Fiber

INGREDIENTS

- 12 ounces canned artichoke hearts, drained
- 1/2 pound cream cheese
- 1/2 cup Cheddar cheese, shredded
- 1/2 cup mayonnaise
- 1 teaspoon garlic, minced
- 4 tablespoons chives
- 2 tablespoons spring onions
- Salt and black pepper, to taste
- 1 teaspoon cayenne pepper

DIRECTIONS

1. In a deep saucepan, combine artichoke hearts and cream cheese over the lowest heat. Let the cheese melt for a couple of minutes.
2. Remove from the heat and add in the remaining

Nutritional Info per Serving:.

3. Taste and adjust the seasonings.
4. Storing
5. Place the cheese and artichoke dip in an airtight container and keep in your refrigerator for 3 to 4 days. Enjoy!

05. Sardine Stuffed-Eggs

Preparation Time: 20 minutes

Servings 6

NUTRITION: 216 Calories; 17.3g Fat; 1.8g Carbs; 12.2g Protein; 0.2g Fiber

INGREDIENTS

- 1 can sardines, drained
- 1/2 teaspoon smoked paprika
- 1 teaspoon fresh or dried basil
- 1 tablespoon fresh chives, chopped
- 1 poblano pepper, minced
- 12 eggs
- 1/3 cup aioli
- Salt and pepper, to taste

DIRECTIONS

1. Place the eggs in a saucepan and cover them with water by 1 inch. Cover and bring the water to a boil over high heat. Boil for 6 to 7 minutes over medium- high heat.

2. Peel the eggs and slice them in half lengthwise; mix the yolks with the remaining Ingredients.
3. Divide the mixture among the egg whites.
4. Storing
5. Place the deviled eggs in an airtight container or Ziploc bag; transfer to your refrigerator; they should be consumed within 2 days.
6. For freezing, spoon out the yolk mixture from the deviled eggs. Add the egg yolk mixture to an airtight container or Ziploc bag.
7. Place the container in the freezer for up to 3 months. To defrost, let them sit overnight in the refrigerator until they are fully thawed out. Enjoy!

06. Chicken Wings with Cheese Dip

Preparation Time: 1 hour 15 minutes

Servings 10

NUTRITION: 227 Calories; 10.2g Fat; 0.4g Carbs; 31.5g Protein; 0.2g Fiber

INGREDIENTS

- 3 pounds chicken wings
- Salt and red pepper, to taste
- 1 teaspoon mustard seeds
- 1 teaspoon olive oil

For Feta Cheese Dip:

- 2 tablespoons sour cream
- 1/4 cup fresh parsley leaves, finely chopped
- 2 cloves garlic, smashed
- 1 teaspoon porcini powder
- 1/2 teaspoon ground cumin
- 1 cup feta cheese, shredded
- 1/3 cup mayonnaise

DIRECTIONS

1. Toss the chicken wings with the olive oil, salt, red pepper, and mustard seeds.
2. Roast in the preheated oven at 380 degrees F approximately 35 minutes.
3. Turn the oven up to 410 degrees F and bake for a further 35 minutes on the higher shelf until crispy.
4. In the meantime, mix all Nutritional Info per Serving: for the cheese sauce.
5. Storing
6. Place the chicken wings in airtight containers or Ziploc bags; keep in your refrigerator for up 3 to 4 days.
7. For freezing, place the chicken wings in airtight containers or heavy-duty freezer bags. Freeze up to 3 months. Once thawed in the refrigerator, heat in the preheated oven at 375 degrees F for 20 to 25 minutes or until heated through.
8. Place the feta cheese dip in a glass jar with an airtight lid; keep in your refrigerator for 3 to 4 days. Enjoy!

07. Celery Fries with Pecans

Preparation Time: 35 minutes

Servings 6

NUTRITION: 96 Calories; 8.5g Fat; 4.1g Carbs; 1.5g Protein; 2.6g Fiber

INGREDIENTS

- 1 ½ pounds celery root, cut into sticks
- 2 tablespoons sesame oil
- 1/4 cup pecans, coarsely ground
- 1 tablespoon Adobo seasoning mix
- Salt and pepper, to taste
- 1/2 teaspoon smoked paprika

DIRECTIONS

1. Start by preheating your oven to 395 degrees F. Coat a baking sheet with a Silpat mat.
2. Toss the celery root with the sesame oil, salt, pepper, paprika, and Adobo seasoning mix.
3. Place the celery stick on the prepared baking sheet

and bake in the preheated oven for 30 to 35 minutes, turning them over once or twice.

4. Sprinkle with pecans.
5. Storing
    6. Place the celery fries in airtight containers or Ziploc bags; keep in your refrigerator for up to 3 to 4 days.
    7. To freeze, place the celery fries in airtight containers or Ziploc bags. Freeze up to 5 months. Defrost in the refrigerator. Bon appétit!

08. Chicharrones with Cream Cheese Dip

Preparation Time: 3 hours 10 minutes

Servings 10

NUTRITION: 420 Calories; 43g Fat; 3.1g Carbs; 5g Protein; 0.8g Fiber

INGREDIENTS

- 1 tablespoon olive oil
- 1 ½ pounds pork skin, trimmed of excess fat
- Sea salt and pepper, to taste
- 12 ounces cream cheese
- 1/2 cup mayonnaise
- 2 cups mustard greens, torn into pieces and steamed
- 1 tablespoon chili paste (sambal
- 1 teaspoon onion powder
- 1 teaspoon granulated garlic
- 1/4 teaspoon mustard powder

DIRECTIONS

1. Toss the pork skin with salt until well coated. Place them on a wire rack over a baking sheet.
2. Bake in the preheated oven at 350 degrees F for

about 3 hours, until skin is completely dried out.

3. Heat the olive oil in a nonstick skillet and can cook your chicharrónes in batches until they puff up, about 5 minutes. Place on a paper towel-lined plate.
4. Meanwhile, parboil the mustard greens for about 7 minutes. Add in the remaining ingredients and mix to combine well.
5. Storing
6. Place the chicharrones in airtight containers or Ziploc bags; keep in your refrigerator for up to a week. Reheat them in the microwave.
7. Place the cream cheese dip in airtight containers or Ziploc bags; keep in your refrigerator for up to 4 days.
8. To freeze, place the chicharrones in in airtight containers or Ziploc bags. Freeze up to 3 months. Defrost in the refrigerator. Bon appétit!

09. Garlic Romano Chicken Wings

Preparation Time: 1 hour 10 minutes

Servings 6

NUTRITION: 312 Calories; 23g Fat; 0.9g Carbs; 24.6g Protein; 0.3g Fiber

INGREDIENTS

- 2 pounds chicken wings, bone-in
- 1 teaspoon hot sauce
- 1 cup Romano cheese, grated
- Salt and black pepper, to taste
- 2 cloves garlic, smashed
- 1 stick butter
- 1 tablespoon champagne vinegar
- 1/2 cup Italian parsley, chopped

DIRECTIONS

1. Line a large rimmed baking sheet with a metal rack.
2. Preheat an oven to 420 degrees F. Set a metal rack on top of a baking sheet.
3. Toss the wings with salt and black pepper. Bake in the preheated oven at 410 degrees F

until golden and crispy, for 45 to 50 minutes.

4. Place the garlic, butter, vinegar and hot sauce in a saucepan; cook over low heat until the sauce has thickened slightly.
5. Remove from the heat and fold in the cheese; toss the wings with the cheese mixture until well coated. Bake an additional 8 minutes and top with parsley.
6. Storing
7. Place the chicken wings in airtight containers or Ziploc bags; keep in your refrigerator for up 3 to 4 days.
8. For freezing, place the chicken wings in airtight containers or heavy-duty freezer bags. Freeze up to 3 months. Once thawed in the refrigerator, heat in the preheated oven at 375 degrees F for 20 to 25 minutes or until heated through. Enjoy!

10. Bacon and Broccoli Mini Frittatas

Preparation Time: 30 minutes Servings 6

NUTRITION: 375 Calories; 27.6g Fat; 6g Carbs; 24.8g Protein; 1.6g Fiber

INGREDIENTS

- 6 eggs, whisked
- 5 ounces cooked bacon, chopped
- 1 ½ cups cheddar cheese, freshly grated
- 1 head broccoli, grated
- 1 cup onions, chopped
- Sea salt and pepper, to taste
- 1/2 teaspoon Adobo seasoning mix

For the Dipping Sauce:

- 1 Spanish pepper, chopped
- 2 vine-ripened tomatoes, chopped
- 1/2 teaspoon garlic, chopped
- 1/2 shallot, minced
- 2 tablespoons sesame oil
- 1 teaspoon basil

DIRECTIONS

1. In a mixing bowl, combine the eggs, bacon, cheese, broccoli, onions, salt, pepper, and Adobo seasoning mix.
2. Preheat your oven to 385 degrees F.
3. Spoon the mixture into lightly buttered muffin cups and bake for 20 to 30 minutes, or until golden brown.
4. In the meantime, place all the sauce Nutritional Info per Serving: in a saucepan over medium-low heat. Let it simmer until reduced by half.
5. Storing
6. Place the mini frittatas in an airtight container and keep in your refrigerator for 3 to 4 days.
7. Place the tomato sauce in an airtight container and keep in your refrigerator for up to 3 days.
8. To freeze, place the mini frittatas in separate Ziploc bags and freeze up to 3 months. To defrost, place in your microwave for a few minutes.

To freeze, place the tomato sauce in separate Ziploc bags and freeze up to 3 months

DESSERTS

01. Turmeric Milk Latte

Preparation Time: 5 minutes

Cooking Time: 5 minutes

Servings: 1

INGREDIENTS

- 1 cup unsweetened almond milk
- 1 1/2 tsp vanilla
- 1/2 tsp ground cinnamon
- 1/2 tsp ground ginger
- 1 tsp ground turmeric
- 2 tsp MCT oil

DIRECTIONS

1. Heat almond milk in a saucepan over medium heat until just warm. Remove from heat and let it cool for 2-3 minutes.
2. Transfer milk into the blender along with remaining Ingredients and blend until frothy.
3. Serve and enjoy.

NUTRITION:
Calories 139
Fat 13.1g

Carbohydrates 5.8 g

Sugar 0.9 g

Protein 1.3 g

Cholesterol 0 mg

02. Pumpkin Frappuccino

Preparation Time: 5 minutes

Cooking Time: 5 minutes

Servings: 1

INGREDIENTS

- 1 cup unsweetened almond milk
- 1/2 tsp vanilla
- 1/2 tsp pumpkin pie spice
- 1/3 cup pumpkin
    - 1 cup coffee
    - 1 cup ice

DIRECTIONS

1. Add all Ingredients into the blender and blend until smooth.
2. Serve and enjoy.

NUTRITION:

Calories 76 Fat 3.8 g Carbohydrates 8.9 g

Sugar 3 g Protein 2.2 g Cholesterol 0 mg

03. Coconut Mocha

Preparation Time: 5 minutes

Cooking Time: 5 minutes

Servings: 1

INGREDIENTS

- 1/2 cup brewed coffee
- 5 drops liquid stevia
- 1 tbsp coconut butter
- 2 tsp unsweetened cocoa powder
- 2/3 cup unsweetened coconut milk

DIRECTIONS

1. Add all Ingredients into the saucepan and heat over medium-low heat.
2. Whisk until well combined.
3. Serve and enjoy.

NUTRITION: Calories 470, Fat 47.7g Carbohydrates 14.3 g Sugar 6.4 g Protein 5.5 g Cholesterol 0 mg

04. Cinnamon Coffee

Preparation Time: 5 minutes

Cooking Time: 5 minutes

Servings: 2

INGREDIENTS

- 2 cups brewed coffee
- 1 tsp ground cinnamon
- 1 scoop MCT powder
- 2 tbsp butter

DIRECTIONS

1. Add all Ingredients into the blender and blend until frothy.
2. Serve and enjoy.

NUTRITION:

Calories 157, Fat14.4g

Carbohydrates 6 g ,Sugar 0 g ,Protein 1.9 g,

Cholesterol 31 mg

05. Thick & Creamy Pumpkin Shake

Preparation Time: 5 minutes Cooking

Time: 5 minutes

Servings: 1

INGREDIENTS

- 1 cup unsweetened almond milk
- 5 drops liquid stevia
- 1 tsp cinnamon
- 1/2 tsp pumpkin spice
- 1 tsp vanilla
- 2 tbsp heavy cream
- 3 tbsp pumpkin puree
- 2 oz cream cheese
- 1/2 cup ice

DIRECTIONS

1. Add all Ingredients into the blender and blend until smooth.
2. Serve and enjoy.

NUTRITION: Calories378, Fat34.6g

Carbohydrates 11 g Sugar 2.3 g Protein 6.6 g

Cholesterol 103 mg

06. Chocolate Pops

Preparation Time: 5 minutes

Cooking Time: 5 minutes

Servings: 6

INGREDIENTS

- 4 oz unsweetened chocolate, chopped
- 1 1/2 cup heavy cream
- 6 drops liquid stevia

DIRECTIONS

1. Add heavy cream in a saucepan and heat over medium heat until it just begins to boil.
2. Remove from heat. Add chopped chocolate into the heavy cream and stir well. Let it sit for 5 minutes.
3. Add sweetener and whisk until chocolate is melted.
4. Pour into the popsicle molds and place into the refrigerator until set.
5. Serve and enjoy.

NUTRITION:

Calories 295

Fat 29.9g

Carbohydrates 5.6 g

Sugar 0.2 g

Protein 2.4 g

Cholesterol 80 mg

07. Lime Strawberry Pops

Preparation Time: 5 minutes

Cooking Time: 5 minutes

Servings: 4

INGREDIENTS

- 10 fresh strawberries
- 1 tbsp swerve
- 2 tbsp water
- 1 lime juice

DIRECTIONS

1. Add all Ingredients into the blender and blend until smooth.
2. Pour into the popsicle molds and place into the refrigerator until set.
3. Serve and enjoy.

NUTRITION: Calories 14 Fat 0.1 g Carbohydrates 3.7 g Sugar 1.7 g Protein 0.2 g Cholesterol 0 mg

08. Coconut Strawberry Pops

Preparation Time: 5 minutes Cooking

Time: 5 minutes

Servings: 6

INGREDIENTS

- 14 oz coconut cream
- 1/2 tsp vanilla
- 1/4 cup unsweetened flaked coconut
- 1/4 cup Swerve
- 1 cup heavy whipping cream
- 1 1/2 cups fresh strawberries, chopped

DIRECTIONS

4. Add coconut cream, vanilla, swerve, whipping cream, and strawberries into the food processor and process until smooth.
5. Add flaked coconut and stir well.
6. Pour into the popsicle molds and place into the refrigerator until set.
7. Serve and enjoy.

NUTRITION:

Calories 246

Fat 24.4g

Carbohydrates 7.6 g

Sugar 4.2 g

Protein 2.3 g

Cholesterol 27 mg

09. Greek-Style Coconut Cheesecake

Preparation Time: 30 minutes

Servings 12

NUTRITION: 246 Calories; 22.2g Fat; 5.7g Carbs; 8.1g Protein; 1.9g Fiber

INGREDIENTS

- 5 ounces Greek-style yogurt
- 1 ounce coconut flakes
- 10 ounces almond meal
- 1/4 teaspoon grated nutmeg
- 1 teaspoon lemon zest
- 5 ounces soft cheese
- 1 teaspoon baking powder
- 4 eggs, lightly beaten
- 4 ounces Swerve
- 1/4 coconut oil

DIRECTIONS

1. Brush two spring form pans with a nonstick spray.
2. Mix the almond meal, coconut flakes, nutmeg, and baking powder. Add in the eggs, one at a time, whisking constantly; add in 2 ounces of

Swerve.

3. Spoon the mixture into spring form pans and bake at 360 degrees F for 23 minutes.
4. In another bowl, combine the coconut oil, lemon zest, yogurt, soft cheese, and the remaining 2 ounces of Swerve. Mix to combine and spoon the filling over the first crust. Spread half of the filling over it.
5. Top with another crust and spread the rest of the filling over the top.
6. Storing

7. Place your cheesecake in airtight containers and refrigerate for a week.
8. To freeze, place your cheesecake on a baking tray and freeze for 2 hours. Now, place them in airtight containers. They can be frozen for 2 to 3 months. Bon appétit!

10. Butterscotch Cheesecake Cupcakes

Preparation Time: 30 minutes + chilling time Servings 8

NUTRITION: 165 Calories; 15.6g Fat; 5.4g Carbs; 5.2g Protein; 1.7g Fiber

INGREDIENTS

- 2 eggs
- 1 tablespoon whiskey
- 2 packets stevia
- 3 tablespoons butter, melted
- 10 ounces soft cheese, at room temperature
- 1/2 teaspoon ground cinnamon
- For the Frosting:
- 1 teaspoon butterscotch extract
- 1/2 stick butter, at room temperature
- 1/2 cup powdered erythritol
- 1 ½ tablespoons coconut milk, unsweetened

DIRECTIONS

1. Start by preheating your oven to 365 degrees f.
2. Mix 3 tablespoons of butter, soft cheese, whiskey, eggs, stevia, and cinnamon until well combined.

3. Scrape the batter into the muffin pan and bake approximately 15 minutes; place the muffin pan in the freezer for 2 hours.
4. In a mixing bowl, beat 1/2 stick of butter with powdered erythritol and butterscotch extract.
5. Gradually pour in the milk and mix again. Afterwards, frost the chilled cupcakes.
6. Storing
7. Place your cupcakes in airtight containers and refrigerate for a week.
8. To freeze, place your cupcakes on a baking tray and freeze for 2 hours. Now, place them in airtight containers. They can be frozen for 2 to 3 months. Bon appétit!

11. The Best Keto Birthday Cake

Preparation Time: 40 minutes + chilling time

Servings 10

NUTRITION: 241 Calories; 22.6g Fat; 4.2g Carbs; 6.6g Protein; 0.7g Fiber

INGREDIENTS

- For the Cake Base:
- 2/3 cup coconut flour
- 2 ½ tablespoons butter
- 4 eggs
- 1 cup full-fat milk
- 1 teaspoon vanilla extract
- 1 ½ cups almond meal
- 1/2 teaspoon baking powder
- A pinch of coarse salt
- 1 cup erythritol
- For the Frosting:
- 1/3 cup erythritol
- 3 ounces coconut oil, at room temperature
- A few drops coconut flavor

- 10 ounces soft cheese

DIRECTIONS

1. Mix all Ingredients for the cake base until well combined.
2. Press the crust into a parchment-lined springform pan. Bake at 365 degrees F for 30 minutes or until a toothpick comes outclean; allow it to cool to room temperature.
3. Meanwhile, beat the cheese using your electric mixer until creamy. Stir in the remaining Ingredients and continue to mix until well combined.
4. Frost your cake and serve well-chilled.
5. Storing
6. Place your cheesecake in airtight containers and refrigerate for a week.
7. To freeze, place your cheesecake on a baking tray and freeze for 2 hours. Now, place them in airtight containers. They can be frozen for 2 to 3 months. Bon appétit!

12. Tangerine Chocolate Pudding

Preparation Time: 15 minutes + chilling time

Servings 6

NUTRITION: 158 Calories; 15.7g Fat; 7.2g Carbs; 2.2g Protein; 1.6g Fiber

INGREDIENTS

- 3 1/3 tablespoons Dutch-processed brown cocoa powder
- 2 cups whipped cream
- Fresh juice and zest of 1/2 tangerine
- 1/4 teaspoon ground cloves
- 1/2 teaspoon crystallized ginger
- 6 ounces chocolate, unsweetened
- 3 tablespoons powdered erythritol

DIRECTIONS

1. Using a stand mixer with a whisk attachment, whip the cream until soft peaks form.
2. Add in the powdered erythritol and cocoa powder and beat again. Add in the remaining Ingredients and beat until everything is well incorporated.

3. Storing
4. Spoon your pudding into six airtight containers; keep in your refrigerator for 5 to 6 days.
5. To freeze, place your pudding in six airtight containers; freeze up to 1 month.

13. Peanut Butter Mousse

Preparation Time: 15 minutes
Servings 4

NUTRITION: 288 Calories; 27.3g Fat; 6.9g Carbs; 6.2g Protein; 5.2g Fiber

INGREDIENTS

- 1/2 cup peanut butter
- 1 ½ cups avocado, peeled, pitted, and diced
- 1 teaspoon vanilla extract
- 1 tablespoon lemon juice
- 1/2 cup coconut cream
- 1 teaspoon monk fruit powder
- 1/2 cup coconut milk

DIRECTIONS

1. Place all Ingredients in your blender or food processor. Process until well combined.
2. Storing
3. Spoon your mousse into four airtight containers; keep in your refrigerator for 5 to 6 days.

14. Decadent Macchiato Penuche

Preparation Time: 10 minutes + chilling time

Servings 8

NUTRITION: 145 Calories; 12.8g Fat; 6.2g Carbs; 0.9g Protein; 1.2g Fiber

INGREDIENTS

- 1 teaspoon warm coffee
- 1 teaspoon caramel flavor
- 6 tablespoons butter
- 1 tablespoon peanut butter
- 3 ounces dark chocolate, unsweetened
- 1 teaspoon liquid Monk fruit

DIRECTIONS

1. Microwave the butter and chocolate until they are completely melted.
2. Fold in the remaining Ingredients. Spoon the batter into a foil-lined baking pan, smoothing out the top.
3. Place in your refrigerator for 30 minutes before cutting.
4. Storing

5. Cover your penuche with foil or plastic wrap to prevent drying out; keep in your refrigerator for a week.
6. To freeze, wrap your penuche tightly with foil or place in a heavy-duty freezer bag. Freeze for up to 4 to 6 months. Enjoy!

CONCLUSION

We hope that this cookbook has met your expectations and that you enjoyed yourself in the kitchen! Have you tried all the tasty dishes we have included? What were your favorites? Remember that you can always repeat the recipes by applying personal changes, cooking is a real art and you can customize the dishes to your liking! If you liked this book, recommend it to a friend so that you can have fun with a real challenge to the best and most original dish.

Enjoy your meal!!

CPSIA information can be obtained
at www.ICGtesting.com
Printed in the USA
LVHW020356010221
677957LV00006BA/225

9 781801 595698